For:

PAPA GUARNEI.

"TO MEASURE THE MAN
MEASURE HIS HEART"
        Malcolm S. Forber

To my Father In Law
who has the Largest and
Most Generous Heart I
Know. A MAN I Respect
AND LOVE.

                LOVE,
                    Sherman

Healing
Wisdom

DUTTON
Published by the Penguin Group
Penguin Books USA Inc., 375 Hudson Street,
New York, New York 10014, U.S.A.
Penguin Books Ltd, 27 Wrights Lane, London W8 5TZ, England
Penguin Books Australia Ltd, Ringwood, Victoria, Australia
Penguin Books Canada Ltd, 10 Alcorn Avenue, Toronto, Ontario, Canada M4V 3B2
Penguin Books (N.Z.) Ltd, 182–190 Wairau Road,
Auckland 10, New Zealand

Penguin Books Ltd, Registered Offices: Harmondsworth, Middlesex, England

First published by Dutton, an imprint of Dutton Signet,
a division of Penguin Books USA Inc.
Distributed in Canada by McClelland & Stewart Inc.

First Printing, July, 1994
10 9 8 7 6 5 4 3 2 1

NOTE: The ideas and suggestions contained in this book are not intended as a substitute for consulting with your physician. All matters regarding your health require medical supervision.

Library of Congress Cataloging-in-Publication Data
Anderson, Greg, 1947–
    Healing wisdom : 500 pearls of wit, insight & inspiration for
anyone facing illness / by Greg Anderson.
        p.   cm.
    ISBN 0-525-93774-9
    1. Healing—Quotations, maxims, etc.   2. Medicine—Quotations,
maxims, etc.   I. Title.
RA776.5.A63   1994
610—dc20   94-2711
                                                            CIP

Printed in the United States of America
Set in Goudy Old Style
Designed by Eve L. Kirch

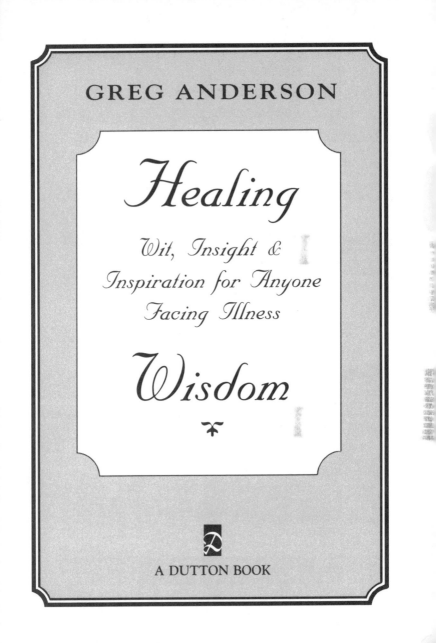

GREG ANDERSON

Healing

Wit, Insight &
Inspiration for Anyone
Facing Illness

Wisdom

A DUTTON BOOK

To all who seek healing, look within.

And to my wife, Linda, and our daughter,
Erica, who fill my life with love.

Acknowledgments

A sincere thank-you to the many people who brought their talent and wisdom to this project. It was a labor of love.

Special thanks to Audrey LaFehr, who makes editing an art form, and to my literary agent, Richard Curtis, who helps me make sense of this business.

And thank you, God, for healing, for new life and real hope when I thought there was none.

Contents

✦

Introduction

✣

It took ten years to compile this book. I began in 1984 after having been diagnosed with lung cancer. I became deeply despondent and depressed. Four months after the initial diagnosis, a second surgery determined I now had cancer throughout the lymph system. My doctor went on to tell me there was nothing more he could do and that I had about thirty days to live.

Even though I was mired in despair, I wanted to do all I could to help myself get well again. I developed a voracious appetite for healing knowledge. I started to read and study. As I did, I would write down and reflect on the most vivid and important points.

Over the years, I have amassed a library on virtually all aspects of healing. I've kept writing down the key thoughts and affirmations on scraps of paper and in my wellness notebook. Now I have gathered this collection of favorite healing words into this little volume. Its purpose is simple: to deliver you a word of hope.

I know that the times of despair, confusion, pain, frustration, and suffering associated with life-threatening illness are many. But I also believe that you and I are capable of personally demonstrating the promise of self-healing in body, mind, and spirit.

Contemplate the truths in these pages. As you read, ask yourself, "How does this apply in my own healing journey?" I trust that through these words of hope you will tap your own God-given healing capabilities, draw strength when you need it, and become determined to live your life to the fullest no matter what the circumstances.

Every once in a while, life hands us a problem that seems overwhelming. If illness seems that way to you, make this book your companion. Read. Reflect. Respond. I know that you, too, can benefit from the great healing wisdom of the ages.

Learn to listen carefully.
Healing wisdom knocks softly.
—GREG ANDERSON

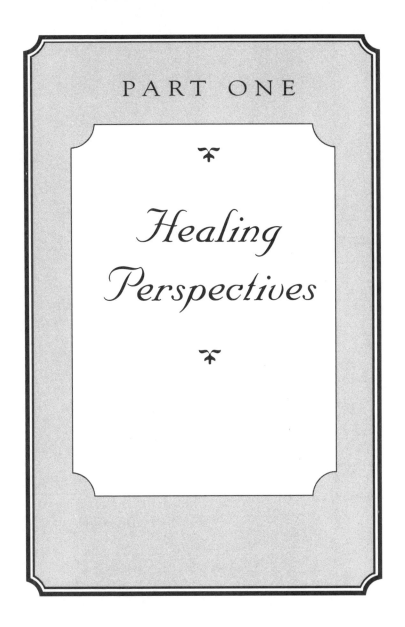

PART ONE

Healing

Perspectives

Natural forces are the healers of disease.

—HIPPOCRATES

✲

Although the world is full of suffering, it is also full of the overcoming of it.

—HELEN KELLER

✲

Faith is the bird that sings while it is still dark.

—ANONYMOUS

✲

The woods would be very quiet if no birds sang there except those who sang best.

—JOHN AUDUBON

✲

The strength you've insisted on assigning to others is actually within yourself.

—LISA ALTHER

✲

Let us then be up and doing, with a heart for any fate.

—HENRY WADSWORTH LONGFELLOW

Honor your challenges, for those spaces that you label as dark are actually there to bring you more light. —SANAYA ROMAN

✺

The biological chain that holds our parts together is only as strong as the weakest vital link. —HANS SELYE

✺

Illness is the doctor to whom we pay most heed; to kindness, to knowledge, we make promises only; to pain we obey.

—MARCEL PROUST

✺

The dark or sick days need not be seen as bad days, for they often prompt our deepest reflection and, in some cases, a change of lifestyle. In this sense, then, one can look upon darkness or disease not as an end but as a beginning of growth.

—EILEEN ROCKEFELLER GROWALD

✺

Despise no new accident in your body, but ask opinion of it. —FRANCIS BACON

❧

Suffering presents us with a challenge: to find goals and purpose in our lives that make even the situation worth living through.

—VIKTOR FRANKL

❧

Pain is part of being alive, and we need to learn that pain does not last forever, nor is it necessarily unbearable, and we need to be taught that. —HAROLD KUSHNER

❧

Ponder the remarkable life force possessed by the body, the body's ability to heal its own wounds and mend its broken bones, indeed, the very wisdom shown by the body.

—RICHARD DeROECK

❧

Perhaps the grandest power of health is self-healing. I say "grandest" because it's the least expensive, most accessible, and, in some ways, the most potent of health forces. It's inexpensive because your body supplies it free. It's accessible because it's part of you. It's potent because through the immune defenses it can slay germs by the millions, repel countless ills, avert a hundred microscopic calamities.

—ROBERT RODALE

What we call disease is nothing more than the body's own effort to cleanse itself of toxins.

—JOHN HENRY TILDEN

Ultimately, we will be healthier, not because of new drugs or surgical techniques, but because of the things we will do for ourselves.

—LOUIS SULLIVAN

All acts of healing are ultimately our selves healing our Self.   —RAM DASS

People are healed by different kinds of healers and systems because the real healer is within.
—GEORGE GOODHEART

Early to bed and early to rise,
makes a man healthy, wealthy, and wise.
—BENJAMIN FRANKLIN

The next major advance in the health of the American people will result only from what the individual is willing to do for himself.
—JOHN KNOWLES

The medical school of the future will concentrate its efforts upon bringing about that harmony between body, mind, and soul which results in the relief and cure of disease.
—EDWARD BACH

Nature, time, and patience are the three great physicians. —CHINESE PROVERB

Nothing in excess. —TEMPLE AT DELPHI

I learned that nothing is impossible when we follow our inner guidance, even when its direction may threaten us by reversing our usual logic. —GERALD JAMPOLSKY

The essence of optimism is that it . . . enables a man to hold his head high, to claim the future for himself and not abandon it to his enemy. —DIETRICH BONHOEFFER

It is not the mountain we conquer but ourselves. —SIR EDMUND HILLARY

Measure your health by your sympathy with morning and spring. If there is no response in you to the awakening of nature, if the prospect of an early morning walk does not banish sleep, if the warble of the first bluebird does not thrill you, know that the morning and spring of your life are past. Thus may you measure your pulse.

—HENRY DAVID THOREAU

✷

It is wisdom to believe the heart.

—GEORGE SANTAYANA

✷

It is not death or pain that is to be dreaded, but the fear of pain or death.   —EPICTETUS

✷

We are never as fortunate or as unfortunate as we suppose.   —LA ROCHEFOUCAULD

✷

Every calamity is a spur and a valuable hint.

—RALPH WALDO EMERSON

✷

Self-pity is our worst enemy, and if we yield to it, we can never do anything wise in this world. —HELEN KELLER

✵

A man too busy to take care of his health is like a lover too busy to care for his mistress— troubled. —SPANISH PROVERB

✵

He who conceals his disease cannot expect to be cured. —ETHIOPIAN PROVERB

✵

Do not be sick. The sick man is more than half a rascal. He may only be sick because he hasn't the courage to clean house. Many sick people are bullies—they use sickness as a club to beat others. —SHERWOOD ANDERSON

✵

Tough times never last; tough people do. —ROBERT H. SCHULLER

✵

How a person masters his fate is more important than what his fate is.

—Wilhelm von Humboldt

✾

Look well into thyself; there is a source of strength which will always spring up if thou wilt always look there.

—Marcus Aurelius

✾

Sometimes what we think is so impossible turns out to be possible after all.

—K. O'Brien

✾

Disease can be healed, if we are willing to change the way we think and believe and act.

—Louise Hay

Happiness is contagious. Be a carrier!
—ROBERT ORBEN

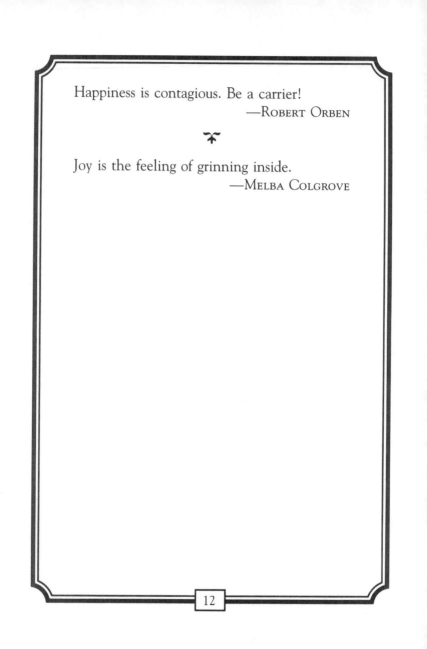

Joy is the feeling of grinning inside.
—MELBA COLGROVE

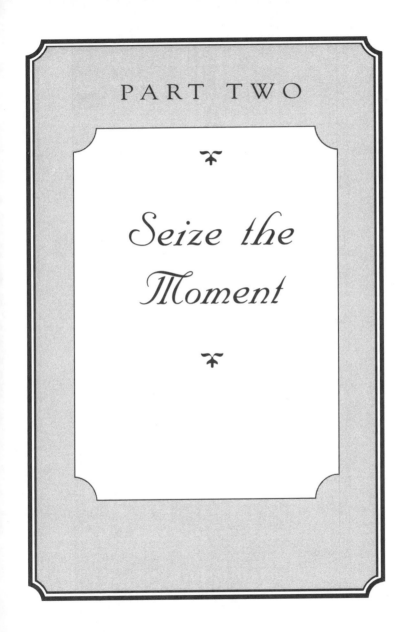

PART TWO

Seize the
Moment

Dare to be wise; begin! He who postpones the hour of living rightly is like the rustic who waits for the river to run out before he crosses.

—HORACE

🦋

Life is a great and wondrous mystery, and the only thing we know that we have for sure is what is right here right now. Don't miss it.

—LEO F. BUSCAGLIA

🦋

It's not too late. —ANONYMOUS

🦋

When you get into a tight place, and everything goes against you till it seems as though you could not hold on a moment longer, never give up then, for that is just the place and time that the tide will turn.

—HARRIET BEECHER STOWE

🦋

It ain't over till it's over. —YOGI BERRA

🦋

Lose an hour in the morning and you will spend all day looking for it.

—RICHARD WHATLEY

🦅

One crowded hour of glorious life is worth an age without a name.

—THOMAS OSBERT MORDAUNT

🦅

One always has time enough, if only one applies it well.　　　　—GOETHE

🦅

Life is a succession of moments. To live each one is to succeed.　　　—CORITA KENT

🦅

Life is uncharted territory. It reveals its story one moment at a time.　—LEO F. BUSCAGLIA

🦅

Live and make the present hour cheerful.
                                    —JOHN A. SCHINDLER

☙

I recommend you to take care of the minutes,
for the hours will take care of themselves.
        —P. D. STANHOPE, EARL OF CHESTERFIELD

☙

And if not now, when?   —THE TALMUD

☙

The ideal day never comes. Today is ideal for
him who makes it so.
                                    —HORATIO W. DRESSER

☙

You learn to build your roads on today, because tomorrow's ground is too uncertain for
plans, and futures have a way of falling down
in midflight.   —VERONICA SHOFFSTAL

☙

Some there are that torment themselves afresh with many memories of what is past; others, again, afflict themselves with the appreciation of evils to come; and very ridiculously—for one does not now concern us, and the other not yet. . . . One should count each day a separate life. —SENECA

There will come a time when you believe everything is finished. That will be the beginning. —LOUIS L'AMOUR

There is no journey to healing. Healing is the journey. —GREG ANDERSON

Most of us spend fifty-nine minutes in an hour living in the past with regret for lost joys, or shame for things badly done . . . or in a future which we either long for or dread.

—STORM JAMESON

One day at a time—
        this is enough
Do not look back
        and grieve over the past,
        for it is gone;
And do not be troubled
        about the future,
        for it has not yet come.
Live in the present,
        and make it so beautiful
        that it will be worth
        remembering.
                —IDA SCOTT TAYLOR

❧

The bridges you cross before you come to them are over rivers that aren't there.
                —GENE BROWN

❧

There are two days about which nobody should ever worry, and these are yesterday and tomorrow.   —ROBERT J. BURDETTE

❧

Yesterday is a canceled check; tomorrow is a promissory note; today is the only cash you have—so spend it wisely.　　—KAY LYONS

※

The only way to ensure a good future is to maximize the present. Focus on the present. Make the present good.

—MARILYN DIAMOND

※

What next? Why ask? Next will come a demand about which you already know all you need to know; that its sole measure is your own strength.　　—DAG HAMMARSKJÖLD

※

One of the tragic things I know about human nature is that all of us tend to put off living. We are all dreaming of some magical rose garden over the horizon—instead of enjoying the roses that are blooming outside our windows today.　　—DALE CARNEGIE

※

Leave tomorrow till tomorrow.

—GERMAN PROVERB

❧

The best thing about the future is that it comes only one day at a time.

—ABRAHAM LINCOLN

❧

Nothing is worth more than this day.

—GOETHE

❧

There is no time like the pleasant.

—OLIVER HERFORD

❧

The future is called "perhaps," which is the only possible thing to call the future. And the important thing is not to allow that to scare you.   —TENNESSEE WILLIAMS

❧

Worry is the interest paid on trouble before it becomes due.   —WILLIAM RALPH INGE

❧

Tomorrow's life is too late; live today.

—MARTIAL

The passing moment is all that we can be sure of; it is only common sense to extract its utmost value from it; the future will one day be the present and will seem as unimportant as the present does now.

—W. SOMERSET MAUGHAM

Let's have a merry journey, and shout about how light is good and dark is not. What we should do is not *future* ourselves so much. We should *now* ourselves more. "*Now* yourself" is more important than "know yourself."

—MEL BROOKS

You won't achieve wellness by starting tomorrow.

—ANONYMOUS

Each day comes bearing its gifts. Untie the ribbons.

—ANN SCHABACKER

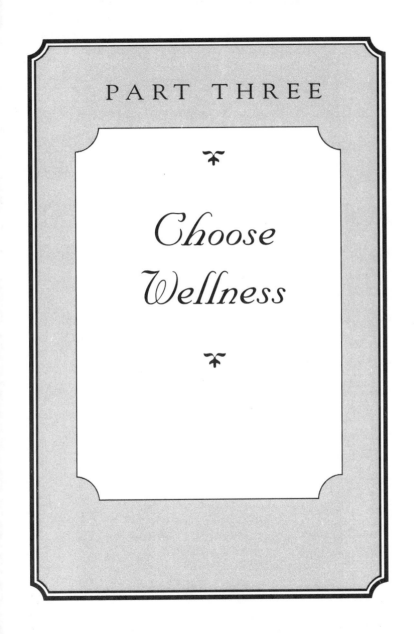

PART THREE

Choose
Wellness

If you are too busy to feel miserable, you will be happy. —ANONYMOUS

When you cannot remove an object, plow around it. But keep plowing.
—MEGIDDO MESSAGE

A man without a plan for the day is lost before he starts. —LEWIS BENDELE

Learning is discovering that something is possible. —FRITZ PERLS

Life is like a game of cards. The hand that is dealt you represents determinism; the way you play it is free will. —NEHRU

You gain strength, courage, and confidence by every experience in which you really stop to look fear in the face. You are able to say to yourself, "I lived through this horror. I can take the next thing that comes along." You must do the thing you cannot do.

—ELEANOR ROOSEVELT

✺

If you can't sleep, then get up and do something instead of lying there and worrying. It's the worry that gets you, not the loss of sleep.

—DALE CARNEGIE

✺

Chance favors the prepared mind.

—LOUIS PERLS

✺

We can either change the complexities of life . . . or develop ways that enable us to cope more effectively.   —HERBERT BENSON

✺

When I go into the garden to spade and dig a bed, I feel such exhilaration and health that I discover that I have been defrauding myself all this time in letting others do for me what I should have done with my own hands.

—RALPH WALDO EMERSON

✶

We sit at breakfast, we sit on the train on the way to work, we sit at work, we sit at lunch, we sit all afternoon . . . a hodgepodge of sagging livers, sinking gall bladders, drooping stomachs, compressed intestines, and squashed organs.

—JOHN BUTTON, JR.

✶

"I must do something" will always solve more problems than "something must be done."

—*Bits & Pieces*

✶

The only true happiness comes from squandering ourselves for a purpose.

—WILLIAM COWPER

✶

Setbacks pave the way for comebacks.

—*Prism*

❧

Don't lie down when you can sit. Don't sit when you can stand. Don't stand when you can move. —Laurence E. Morehouse

❧

We lose much by fearing to attempt.

—J. N. Moffit

❧

Believe in yourself! Have faith in your abilities! Without a humble but reasonable confidence in your own powers you cannot be successful or happy. . . . Formulate and stamp indelibly on your mind a mental picture of yourself as succeeding. Hold this picture tenaciously. Never permit it to fade. Your mind will seek to develop this picture. . . .

—Norman Vincent Peale

❧

For they conquer who believe they can.

—Ralph Waldo Emerson

Belief is a potent medicine.
—STEVEN E. LOCKE AND DOUGLAS COLLIGAN

❧

To remain healthy, man must have some goal, some purpose in life that he can respect and be proud to work for.   —HANS SELYE

❧

Those who do not find time for exercise will have to find time for illness.
—OLD PROVERB

❧

Health lies in labor, and there is no royal road to it but through toil.   —WENDELL PHILLIPS

❧

A little labor, much health.
—GEORGE HERBERT

❧

Walking is man's best medicine.
—HIPPOCRATES

❧

Walking makes for a long life.

—HINDU PROVERB

*

It is better to wear out than rust out.

—RICHARD CUMBERLAND

*

The wise, for cure, on exercise depend.

—JOHN DRYDEN

*

There are no gains without pains.

—ADLAI STEVENSON

*

Work is the grand cure for all the maladies and miseries that ever beset mankind—honest work, which you intend getting done.

—THOMAS CARLYLE

*

He who will have no time for health today may have no health for time tomorrow.

—ANONYMOUS

*

No one knows what it is that he can do till he tries.
—Publilius Syrus

❋

To know oneself, one should assert oneself.
—Albert Camus

❋

Life is not always what one wants it to be, but to make the best of it as it is, is the only way of being happy.
—Jennie Jerome Churchill

❋

Just for today—I will live through the next 12 hours and try not to tackle all life's problems at once.
—Alcoholics Anonymous

❋

Don't find fault. Find a remedy.
—Henry Ford

❋

Usually when people are sad, they don't do anything. They just cry over their condition. But when they get angry, they bring about a change. —MALCOLM X

❧

Our remedies oft in ourselves do lie,
Which we ascribe to heaven. —SHAKESPEARE

❧

Prayer is indeed good, but while calling on the gods a man should himself lend a hand.

—HIPPOCRATES

❧

Our prayers are answered not when we are given what we ask, but when we are challenged to be what we can be.

—MORRIS ADLER

❧

Fight one more round. When your feet are so tired you have to shuffle back to the center of the ring, fight one more round.

—JAMES J. CORBETT

❧

Fall seven times, stand up eight.

—JAPANESE PROVERB

❈

When fate knocks you flat on your back, remember she leaves you looking up.

—ANONYMOUS

❈

Before you begin a thing, remind yourself that difficulties and delays quite impossible to foresee are ahead. If you could see them clearly, naturally you could do a great deal to get rid of them but you can't. You can only see one thing clearly and that is your goal. Form a mental vision of that and cling to it through thick and thin.   —KATHLEEN NORRIS

❈

If all difficulties were known at the outset of a long journey, most of us would never start out at all.   —DAN RATHER

❈

The beginning is the most important part of the work.   —PLATO

The journey of a thousand miles begins with one step. —LAO-TZU

❧

No great thing is created suddenly, any more than a bunch of grapes or a fig. If you tell me that you desire a fig, I answer you that there must be time. Let it first blossom, then bear fruit, then ripen. —EPICTETUS

❧

Blessed is he who found his work; let him ask no other blessedness. He has a work, a life purpose; he has found it, and will follow it. —THOMAS CARLYLE

❧

If there is no wind, row. —INDIAN PROVERB

❧

There's always room for improvement—it's the biggest room in the house. —LOUISE HEATH LEBER

❧

The important thing is not to stop questioning. —ALBERT EINSTEIN

There is no failure except in no longer trying.
—ELBERT HUBBARD

This is the true joy in life, the being used for a purpose recognized by yourself as a mighty one. —GEORGE BERNARD SHAW

Your heaviest artillery [in sickness] will be your will to live. Keep that big gun going.
—NORMAN COUSINS

You have to raise yourself above things instead of letting things raise themselves above you.
—JAMES STEPHENS

The great thing in this world is not so much where we are, but in what direction we are going. —OLIVER WENDELL HOLMES

When nothing seems to help, I go and look at a stonecutter hammering away at his rock perhaps a hundred times without as much as a crack showing in it. Yet at the hundred-and-first blow, it will split in two, and I know it was not that blow that did it—but all that had gone before.   —JACOB RIIS

Be not afraid of going slowly, be afraid only of standing still.   —CHINESE PROVERB

Do what you can, with what you have, with where you are.   —THEODORE ROOSEVELT

PART FOUR

Reach
Out

It is one of the most beautiful compensations of this life that no man can sincerely try to help another without helping himself.

—RALPH WALDO EMERSON

❋

The best way to forget your own problems is to help someone else solve his.

—ANONYMOUS

❋

[A] workable and effective way to meet and overcome difficulties is to take on someone else's problems. It is a strange fact, but you can handle two difficulties—your own and somebody else's—better than you can handle your own alone. That truth is based on a subtle law of self-giving or outgoingness whereby you develop a self-strengthening in the process.   —NORMAN VINCENT PEALE

❋

We are not primarily put on this earth to see through one another but to see one another through.   —PETER DE VRIES

❋

A faithful friend is the medicine of life.

—Ecclesiastes

✦

The best cure for worry, depression, melancholy, brooding, is to go deliberately forth and try to lift with one's sympathy the gloom of somebody else. —Arnold Bennett

✦

The greatest object in the universe, says a certain philosopher, is a good man struggling with adversity; yet there is a still greater, which is the good man that comes to relieve it. —Oliver Goldsmith

✦

Help thy brother's boat across, and lo! thine own has reached the shore.

—Hindu proverb

✦

Only the life in service of others is worth living. —Albert Einstein

✦

Disease has social as well as physical, chemical, and biological causes.

—HENRY SIEGRIST

🦅

People are lonely because they build walls instead of bridges.   —JOSEPH FORT NEWTON

🦅

Love received and love given comprise the best form of therapy.   —GORDON ALLPORT

🦅

We all like to forgive, and we all love best not those who offend us least, not those who have done the most for us, but those who make it most easy for us to forgive them.

—SAMUEL BUTLER

🦅

We love persons . . . by reason of their defects as well as of their qualities.

—JACQUES MARITAIN

🦅

Admit your faults to one another and pray for each other so that you may be healed.

—SAINT JAMES

✸

Forgiveness is the answer to the child's dream of a miracle by which what is broken is made whole again, what is soiled is again made clean.

—DAG HAMMARSKJÖLD

✸

To forgive is the highest, most beautiful form of love. In return, you will receive untold peace and happiness.

—ROBERT MULLER

✸

A mental treatment guaranteed to cure every ill that flesh is heir to: sit for half an hour every night and mentally forgive everyone against whom you have any ill will or antipathy.

—CHARLES FILLMORE

✸

The best gift—forgiveness.

—"Dear Abby"

✸

Just for today—I will not find fault with a friend, relative or colleague. I will not try to change or improve anyone but myself.

—ALCOHOLICS ANONYMOUS

※

If you judge people, you have no time to love them. —MOTHER TERESA

※

The joy of life is to put out one's power in some natural and useful or harmless way. There is no other, and the real misery is not to do this. —OLIVER WENDELL HOLMES

※

Do unto others as though you were others.

—ANONYMOUS

※

Keep your fears to yourself, but share your courage with others.

—ROBERT LOUIS STEVENSON

※

People, by and large, will relate to the image you project. . . . If you project the image of a sick dependent person, that's how you'll be treated. —SAMUEL B. CHYATTE

❧

Of all the things you wear, your expression is the most important. —JANET LANE

❧

Illness is telling us what we need to stop doing. It has great value. It forces us to reach out for help, bringing more love to us.
—O. CARL SIMONTON

❧

When one is out of touch with oneself, one cannot touch others. —ANONYMOUS

❧

What do we live for if it is not to make life less difficult for each other?
—GEORGE ELIOT

❧

When you handle yourself, use your head; when you handle others, use your heart.

—DONNA REED

❧

The common denominator of all healing methods is unconditional love—a love that respects the uniqueness of each individual and empowers each person to take responsibility for his or her own well-being.

—JACK SCHWARTZ

❧

Love is a fruit of all seasons at all times and within the reach of every hand.

—MOTHER TERESA

❧

The type of hug I recommend is the bear hug. Use both arms, face your partner and perform a full embrace.   —DAVID BRESLER

❧

I have been sick and I have found out, only then, how lonely I am. Is it too late?

—EUDORA WELTY

The remedy to physical isolation is being with others. The remedy to spiritual isolation is opening ourselves to the spirit of life and love that exists everywhere. —AMY DEAN

☘

Believe, when you are most unhappy, that there is something for you to do in the world. So long as you can sweeten another's pain, life is not in vain. —HELEN KELLER

☘

There is a direct connection between creative thought and involvement in life and the production of epinephrine by the adrenal gland. When the challenge stops, the supply is turned off; the will to live atrophies.

—NORMAN COUSINS

☘

We make a living by what we get, but we make a life by what we give.

—NORMAN MACEWAN

☘

Duty makes us do things well, but love makes us do them beautifully.   —PHILLIP BROOKS

❅

Out of a sense of duty and a desire to protect a loved one, a vicious cycle of misinterpretation, guesswork, silence, and isolation is initiated.   —NEIL A. FIORE

❅

Our health is not just a matter of what we do for our own bodies but what we do for each other and for the planet.   —LOWELL LEVIN

❅

Fear to do ill, and you need fear nought else.
                    —BENJAMIN FRANKLIN

❅

In the final analysis, we must love in order not to fall ill.   —SIGMUND FREUD

❅

Scatter joy.   —RALPH WALDO EMERSON

PART FIVE

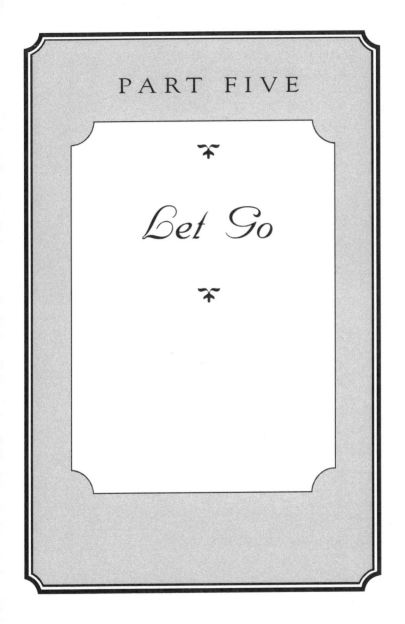

Let Go

Tears are often the telescope through which men see far into heaven.

—Henry Ward Beecher

꙾

Once you have experienced the seriousness of your loss you will be able to experience the wonder of being alive.

—Robert L. Veninga

꙾

Drag your thoughts away from your troubles —by the ears, by the heels, or any other way you can manage it. It's the healthiest thing a body can do.　　　—Mark Twain

꙾

Afflictions are not really a good gift—neither they nor their consequences. However, if afflictions do come, it is well that we convert them into afflictions of love. Herein lies the power of man.　　　—Hayyím Nahman Bialik

꙾

Every life has its dark and cheerful hours. Happiness comes from choosing which to remember. —Anonymous

❦

A pessimist is one who makes difficulties of his opportunities; an optimist makes opportunities of his difficulties.

—Reginald B. Mansell

❦

A pessimist sees the dark side of the clouds, and mopes; a philosopher sees both sides, and shrugs; an optimist doesn't see the clouds at all—he's walking on them.   —D. O. Flynn

❦

No pessimist ever won a battle.

—Dwight D. Eisenhower

❦

Many of life's failures are people who did not realize how close they were to success when they gave up.   —Thomas Edison

❦

Don't be discouraged. It is often the last key in the bunch that opens the lock.

—ANONYMOUS

✦

Look at what you have left, not what you have lost.

—ROBERT H. SCHULLER

✦

Bitterness imprisons life; love releases it.

—HARRY EMERSON FOSDICK

✦

Anger is a wind which blows out the lamp of the mind.

—ROBERT GREEN INGERSOLL

✦

Anger is quieted by a gentle word, just as fire is quenched by water.

—MEGIDDO MESSAGE

✦

When you give vent to your feelings, anger leaves you.

—JEWISH PROVERB

✦

Negative emotions will not harm you if you express them appropriately and then let them go. Bottling them up is far worse.

—JOAN BORYSENKO

✥

Your health is bound to be affected if, day by day, you say the opposite of what you feel, if you grovel before what you dislike, and rejoice at what brings you nothing but misfortune.

—BORIS PASTERNAK

✥

There is perhaps nothing so bad and so dangerous in life as fear.

—NEHRU

✥

Stripped of all their masquerades, the fears of men are quite identical: the fear of loneliness, rejection, inferiority, unmanageable illness and death.

—JOSHUA LOTH LIEBMAN

✥

To hate and to fear is to be psychologically ill. It is, in fact, the consuming illness of our time.

—H. A. OVERSTREET

The strangest and most fantastic fact about negative emotions is that people actually worship them.　　　　　—P. D. OUSPENSKY

＊

A perverse temper and fretful disposition make any state of life whatsoever unhappy.
　　　　　—CICERO

＊

Sadness is almost never anything but a form of fatigue.　　　　　—ANDRÉ GIDE

＊

Troubles, like babies, grow larger by nursing.
　　　　　—ELIZABETH, LADY HOLLAND

＊

To be wronged is nothing unless you continue to remember it.　　　　　—CONFUCIUS

＊

Write injuries in sand, kindnesses in marble.
　　　　　—FRENCH PROVERB

＊

The biggest thing in our today's sorrow is the memory of yesterday's joy.

—Kahlil Gibran

The confrontation with death . . . makes everything look so precious, so sacred, so beautiful, that I feel more strongly than ever the impulse to live it, to embrace it, and to let myself be overwhelmed by it.

—Abraham Maslow

Finish every day and be done with it. You have done what you could. Some blunders and absurdities no doubt crept in; forget them as soon as you can. Tomorrow is a new day; begin it well and serenely and with too high a spirit to be cumbered with your old nonsense. This day is all that is good and fair. It is too dear, with its hopes and invitations, to waste a moment on the yesterdays.

—Ralph Waldo Emerson

How much pain the evils have cost us that have never happened.   —THOMAS JEFFERSON

❦

You should not hold back from making a start because of fears about the future.

—LEWIS PRESNALL

❦

Worry is a thin stream of fear trickling through the mind. If encouraged, it cuts a channel into which all other thoughts are drained.   —ARTHUR SOMERS ROCHE

❦

One hour of worry is one hour of hell.

—JAMES DODDS

❦

The past should be culled like a box of fresh strawberries, rinsed of debris, sweetened judiciously and served in small portions, not very often.   —LAURA PALMER

❦

Learning to let go of negative emotions is the key.   —BERNIE SIEGEL

✼

I believe that all genuine healing addresses the problem of unblocking negatives.

—SUN BEAR

✼

Keep your face to the sunshine and you cannot see the shadow.   —HELEN KELLER

PART SIX

Call on Your Inner Strength

Happiness is not being pained in body nor troubled in mind. —THOMAS JEFFERSON

✺

Don't wait around for other people to be happy for you. Any happiness you get you've got to make yourself. —ABIE WALKER

✺

Most people live, whether physically, intellectually, or morally, in a very restricted circle of their potential being. Great emergencies and crises show us how much greater our vital resources are than we had supposed.

—WILLIAM JAMES

✺

Vitality shows not only in the ability to persist but in the ability to start over.

—F. SCOTT FITZGERALD

✺

Never give in, never, never, never, never.

—WINSTON CHURCHILL

✺

Great souls have wills, feeble ones have wishes.   —CHINESE PROVERB

❋

Consider the postage stamp: its usefulness consists in the ability to stick to one thing till it gets there.   —JOSH BILLINGS

❋

No man is good for anything who has not some particle of obstinacy to use upon occasion.   —HENRY WARD BEECHER

❋

Never consent to creep when you feel an impulse to soar.   —HELEN KELLER

❋

Anger is one of the sinews of the soul; he that wants it hath a maimed mind.

—THOMAS FULLER

❋

Be not afraid of life. Believe that life is worth living, and your belief will help create the fact.

—WILLIAM JAMES

Go fearlessly, not fearfully.   —Anonymous

✼

Patience and fortitude conquer all things.
                    —Ralph Waldo Emerson

✼

We must face what we fear; that is the case
of the core of the restoration of health.
                              —Max Lerner

✼

The only courage that matters is the kind that
gets you from one moment to the next.
                    —Mignon McLaughlin

✼

Courage is not the absence of fear but the
conquest of it.   —Earl Riney

✼

Courage is the fear of being thought a coward.
                            —Horace Smith

✼

Look with thine ears.   —Shakespeare

Curiosity will conquer fear even more than bravery will. —James Stephens

The first thing I had to conquer was fear. I realized what a debilitating thing fear is. It can render you absolutely helpless. I know now that fear breeds fear. —Byron Janis

Positive attitudes—optimism, high self-esteem, an outgoing nature, joyousness, and the ability to cope with stress—when established early in life, may be the most important basis for continued good health. —Helen Hayes

Nothing great was ever achieved without enthusiasm. —Ralph Waldo Emerson

The worst bankrupt is the person who has lost his enthusiasm. —H. W. Arnold

To live is not merely to breathe, it is an act; it is to make use of our organs, senses, faculties, of all those parts of ourselves which give us a feeling of existence.

—Jean-Jacques Rousseau

❧

We can be sure that the greatest hope for maintaining equilibrium in the face of any situation rests within ourselves. Persons who are secure with a transcendental system of values and deep sense of moral duties are possessors of values which no man and no catastrophe can take from him. —Francis Braceland

❧

If a man happens to find himself, he has a mansion which he can inhabit with dignity all the days of his life. —James A. Michener

❧

Always direct your thoughts to those truths that will give you confidence, hope, joy, love, and thanksgiving, and turn away your mind from those that inspire you with fear, sadness, and depression. —Bertrand Wilberforce

Any real progress in the tangled world of emotions must be made by the individual. Each of us must hold the mirror to our own soul and gaze intently at what we see there.

—Bernard S. Raskas

✦

You cannot teach a man anything. You can only help him to find it within himself.

—Galileo

✦

Serenity comes not alone by removing the outward causes and occasions of fear, but by the discovery of inward reservoirs to draw upon. —Rufus M. Jones

✦

In the midst of winter, I finally learned that there was in me an invincible summer.

—Albert Camus

✦

Trust yourself; then you will know how to live. —Goethe

✦

It is the commonest of mistakes to consider that the limit of our power of perception is also the limit of all there is to perceive.
—C. W. Leadbeater

🦅

Paradise is where I am.   —Voltaire

🦅

Write your faults in the sand, your virtues in marble.   —Sister Antonia Brenner

🦅

Above all things, reverence yourself.
—Pythagoras

🦅

Self-love is the instrument of our preservation.
—Voltaire

🦅

Self-love . . . is not so vile a sin as self-neglecting.   —Shakespeare

🦅

The soul is dyed the color of its thoughts.
—MARCUS AURELIUS

The mind is its own place,
and in itself
Can make a heaven of hell,
or a hell of heaven.
—JOHN MILTON

Conscience is a divine voice in the human soul.
—FRANCIS BOWEN

Conscience is a mother-in-law whose visit never ends.
—H. L. MENCKEN

The body mirrors the soul and the mind, and it is much more accessible than either.
—GEORGE SHEEHAN

There can be no happiness if the things we believe in are different from the things we do.
—FREYA STARK

In adversity, man is saved by hope.

—Menander

❧

If we want a joyous life, we must think joyous thoughts. If we want a prosperous life, we must think prosperous thoughts. If we want a loving life, we must think loving thoughts. Whatever we send out mentally or verbally will come back to us in like form.   —Louise Hay

❧

Neither lofty degree of intelligence nor imagination nor both together go to the making of a genius. Love, love, love, that is the soul of genius.   —Mozart

❧

Gratitude is the heart's memory.

—French proverb

❧

Recall it as often as you wish; a happy memory never wears out.   —Libbie Fudim

❧

All healthy things are sweet-tempered.
—RALPH WALDO EMERSON

✼

To live happily is an inward power of the soul.
—MARCUS AURELIUS

✼

There is no difficulty that enough love will not conquer; no disease that enough love will not heal; no door that enough love will not open. . . . It makes no difference how deeply seated may be the trouble; how hopeless the outlook; how muddled the tangle; how great the mistake. A sufficient realization of love will dissolve it all. If only you could love enough you would be the happiest and most powerful being in the world.   —EMMET FOX

✼

Healing is accomplished through love and is love. And love is the uniting principle in all healing approaches.   —HUGH PRATHER

PART SEVEN

Understand Who Heals

The presence of the doctor is the first part of the cure. —FRENCH PROVERB

⋇

The patient must combat the disease along with the physician. —HIPPOCRATES

⋇

When a person is depressed or confused, the physician's advice is just one part of the prescription for spiritual renewal. The patient needs to learn to look within to find his or her own strength. —CARL HAMMERSCHLAG

⋇

The art of medicine consists of amusing the patient while nature cures the disease.
—VOLTAIRE

⋇

After two days in the hospital, I took a turn for the nurse. —W. C. FIELDS

⋇

The placebo makes a statement that we have within us a certain self-regulatory mechanism, a self-healing mechanism, which can be mobilized given proper situational and environmental cues. —DAVID S. SOBEL

✛

Doctors pour drugs of which they know little, to cure diseases of which they know less, into human beings of whom they know nothing.
—VOLTAIRE

✛

Confidence and hope do more good than physic [medicine]. —GALEN

✛

One of the first duties of the physician is to educate the masses not to take medicine.
—SIR WILLIAM OSLER

✛

There ain't much fun in medicine, but there's a heck of a lot of medicine in fun.
—JOSH BILLINGS

✛

I don't see why any man who believes in medicine would shy at the faith cure.

—T. P. Dunne

🕊

He's a devout believer in the department of witchcraft called medical science.

—George Bernard Shaw

🕊

A specialist is one who has his patients trained to become ill only during his office hours. A general practitioner is likely to be called off the golf course at any time.

—*Kansas City Star*

🕊

Surgery is always second best. If you can do something else, it's better.

—John Kirklin, surgeon

🕊

If you think you are ill, call in a doctor. Call in three doctors and play bridge.

—Robert Benchley

🕊

Never go to a doctor whose office plants have died.
—ERMA BOMBECK

🦅

Perfect obedience to the laws of health would abolish the medical profession.
—O. B. FROTHINGHAM

🦅

The cure for many diseases is unknown to the physicians of Hellas, because they are ignorant of the whole, which ought to be studied also; for the part can never be well unless the whole is well.
—PLATO

🦅

Doctors don't understand everything really. They understand matter, not spirit. And you and I live in the spirit.
—WILLIAM SAROYAN

🦅

I firmly believe that if the whole *materia medica*, as now used, could be sunk to the bottom of the sea, it would be all the better for mankind and all the worse for the fishes.

—OLIVER WENDELL HOLMES

The medical profession, because of the public attitude, is made up largely of troubleshooters and repairmen when maintenance men are what are needed most.

—C. C. AND S. M. FURNAS

Everyone should be his own physician. He ought to assist, and not force nature.

—VOLTAIRE

The beginning of health is to know the disease.

—CERVANTES

One of the most common of all diseases is diagnosis.

—KARL KRAUS

We have not lost faith, but we have transferred it from God to the medical profession.
                    —GEORGE BERNARD SHAW

✸

God heals, and the doctor takes the fee.
                    —BENJAMIN FRANKLIN

✸

Who pays the physician does the cure.
                    —GEORGE HERBERT

✸

The purse of the patient protracts his cure.
                    —ANONYMOUS

✸

Money cannot buy health, but I'd settle for a diamond-studded wheelchair.
                    —DOROTHY PARKER

✸

Health is the state about which medicine has nothing to say.   —W. H. AUDEN

✸

It is this intangible thing, love, love in many forms, which enters into every therapeutic relationship. It is an element of which the physician may be the carrier, the vessel. And it is an element which binds and heals, which comforts and restores, which works what we have to call—for now—miracles.

—KARL A. MENNINGER

⋆

There is a wisdom in this beyond the rules of physic [medicine]: a man's own observations, what he finds good of and what he finds hurt of, is the best physic to preserve health.

—FRANCIS BACON

⋆

I take all stories of miraculous healings, spontaneous remissions, and instantaneous cures as evidence for the remarkable self-healing abilities that are possible in all humanity.

—JERRY SOLFVIN

⋆

Nature heals, under the auspices of the medical profession. —HAVEN EMERSON

Some patients, though conscious that their condition is perilous, recover their health simply through their contentment with the goodness of the physician. —HIPPOCRATES

✻

The attitude of the healer is almost as important as the attitude of the person being healed.
—O. CARL SIMONTON

✻

The patient's hopes are the physician's best ally. —NORMAN COUSINS

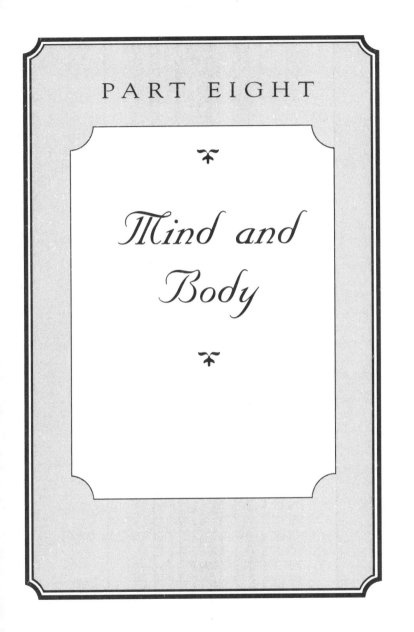

PART EIGHT

Mind and Body

The healing mind is the calm mind.
—GREG ANDERSON

＊

The body is the workhouse of the soul.
—H. G. BOHN

＊

If you are ruled by mind you are a king; if by body, a slave.   —CATO

＊

The more serious the illness, the more important it is for you to fight back, mobilizing all your resources—spiritual, emotional, intellectual, physical.   —NORMAN COUSINS

＊

The fact that the mind rules the body is, in spite of its neglect by biology and medicine, the most fundamental fact which we know about the process of life.
—FRANZ ALEXANDER

＊

If you can get back in tune with your body, it will tell you what it wants. One way of doing that is to start to have more faith and confidence in your own instincts, logic, and common sense. —HARVEY DIAMOND

Coddle the body and you harm the soul.
—POLISH PROVERB

The body is the baggage you must carry through life. The more excess baggage, the shorter the trip. —MARTHA WASHINGTON

Tell me what you eat, and I will tell you what you are. —BRILLAT-SAVARIN

Short supper; long life. —SERBIAN PROVERB

Give up those intimate little dinners for four, unless there are three other people eating with you. —ORSON WELLES

❧

Eat little at night, open windows, drive out often, and look for the good in things and people. . . . You will no longer be sad, or bored, or ill. —MARY KNOWLES

❧

If it grows, eat it. If it doesn't grow, don't eat it. —LOUISE HAY

❧

I have no doubt that it is part of the destiny of the human race, in its gradual improvement, to leave off eating animals, as surely as the savage tribes have left off eating each other when they came in contact with the more civilized. —HENRY DAVID THOREAU

❧

Never eat Chinese food in Oklahoma. —DAVID BRYAN

❧

To avoid illness, eat less. To have a long life, worry less. —CHINESE PROVERB

✦

The physical is the substratum of the spiritual, and this fact ought to give to the food we eat, and the air we breathe, a transcendent significance. —WILLIAM TYNDALE

✦

Just pray for a thick skin and a tender heart. —RUTH BELL GRAHAM

✦

Serious illness doesn't bother me for long because I am too inhospitable a host. —ALBERT SCHWEITZER

✦

The healing process is made up of unconditional love, forgiveness, and letting go of fear. —GERALD JAMPOLSKY

✦

The purpose of healing is to bring us in harmony with ourselves. —O. CARL SIMONTON

Healing does not necessarily mean to become physically well or to be able to get up and walk around again. Rather, it means achieving a balance between the physical, emotional, intellectual, and spiritual dimensions.

—Elisabeth Kübler-Ross

꙳

I'm not OK, you're not OK, and that's OK.

—William Sloane Coffin

꙳

We've discovered that our growth today depends upon our mental, physical, and spiritual health. If we picture these three as the legs of a stool, we can see that shortchanging the importance of one or taking one of them away will upset the balance.   —Amy Dean

꙳

Soul growth is most important of all for developing the highest nature of man. I believe the inner man is most important to take care of.   —Bernard Jensen

꙳

The highest possible stage in moral culture is when we recognize that we ought to control our thoughts. —CHARLES DARWIN

✿

The principal thing in this world is to keep one's soul aloft. —GUSTAVE FLAUBERT

✿

Great men are they who see that spiritual is stronger than any material force, that thoughts rule the world.

—RALPH WALDO EMERSON

✿

The purpose of maintaining the body in good health is to acquire wisdom. —MAIMONIDES

✿

Let us train our minds to desire what the situation demands. —SENECA

✿

Health is not a condition of matter but of mind. —MARY BAKER EDDY

✿

Age is a question of mind over matter. If you don't mind, it doesn't matter.

—SATCHEL PAIGE

✣

I'll tell ya how to stay young; hang around with older people.   —BOB HOPE

✣

Medicine has been blind in thinking that matter is more powerful than mind.

—DEEPAK CHOPRA

✣

The mind has great influence over the body, and maladies often have their origin there.

—MOLIÈRE

✣

Much illness is unhappiness sailing under a physiologic flag.   —RUDOLF VIRCHOW

✣

The best way to cure hypochondria is to forget about your body and get interested in someone else's.   —GOODMAN ACE

Those who see any difference between soul and body have neither.   —OSCAR WILDE

✲

All that we are is a result of what we have thought; it is founded on our thoughts, it is made up of our thoughts. If a man speaks or acts with pure thought, happiness follows him like a shadow that never leaves him.

—BUDDHA

✲

The human body is the best picture of the human soul.   —LUDWIG WITTGENSTEIN

✲

Healing is not a matter of mechanism but a work of the spirit.   —RACHEL NAOMI REMEN

✲

A chronic illness is a constant and sometimes overwhelming companion. . . . Only the power of a warm heart can alleviate the deep chill.   —ROBERT K. MASSIE

✲

A cancer is not only a physical disease, it is a state of mind. —MICHAEL BADEN

✦

Some element in the mind of the patient makes an important difference in the body's reaction to illness, something as ephemeral as an attitude or feeling that could leave its mark on the body.
  —STEVEN E. LOCKE AND DOUGLAS COLLIGAN

✦

To heal the body without including the mind, without allowing the body/mind to sink into the heart, is to continue the grief of a lifetime.
  —STEPHEN LEVINE

✦

A bodily disease which we look upon as whole and entire within itself, may, after all, be but a symptom of some ailment in the spiritual part. —NATHANIEL HAWTHORNE

✦

Happiness should not depend on physical wellness. —K. O'BRIEN

If only we'd stop trying to be happy we'd have a pretty good time.   —EDITH WHARTON

꙳

All you need for happiness is a good gun, a good horse, and a good wife.

—DANIEL BOONE

꙳

So have no fear. Do not fear those who kill the body but cannot kill the soul.

—SAINT MATTHEW

꙳

The natural healing force within each one of us is the greatest force in getting well.

—HIPPOCRATES

꙳

Body and soul cannot be separated for purposes of treatment, for they are one and indivisible.   —C. JEFF MILLER

꙳

One must combine the body, the mind, and the heart—and to keep them in parallel vigor one must exercise, study, and love.

—KARL VON BONSTETTEN

✸

To wish to be well is part of becoming well.

—SENECA

✸

You have to work to make it work.

—ALAN BLUM

✸

Motivation. It's the one part of your health agenda that you can't buy, borrow, or do without. —*Prevention*

✸

Physical strength can never permanently withstand the impact of spiritual force.

—FRANKLIN D. ROOSEVELT

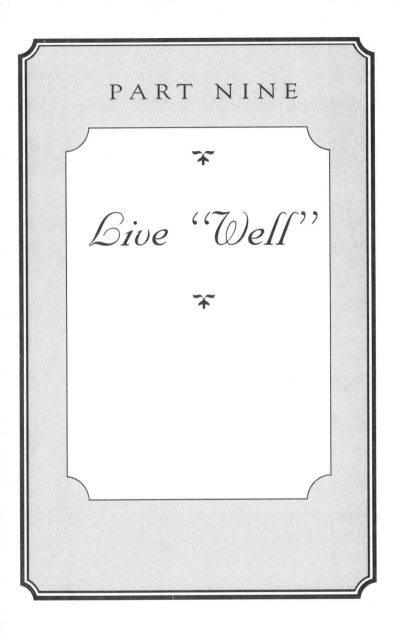

PART NINE

Live "Well"

It matters not how long you live, but how well. —PUBLILIUS SYRUS

✸

Be not afraid of life. Believe that life is worth living and your belief will help create the fact. —WILLIAM JAMES

✸

What we call the secret of happiness is no more a secret than our willingness to choose life. —LEO F. BUSCAGLIA

✸

The fear of death keeps us from living, not from dying. —PAUL C. ROUD

✸

There is no cure for birth and death save to enjoy the interval. —GEORGE SANTAYANA

✸

Do not try to live forever. You will not succeed. —GEORGE BERNARD SHAW

✸

The tragedy of life is not that it ends so soon, but that we wait so long to begin it.
—RICHARD EVANS

✴

Life is not length but depth.   —ANONYMOUS

✴

The real voyage of discovery consists not in seeking new landscapes but in having new eyes.
—MARCEL PROUST

✴

The more passionately we love life, the more intensely we experience the joy of life.
—JÜRGEN MOLTMANN

✴

Try as much as possible to be wholly alive, with all your might, and when you laugh, laugh like hell, and when you get angry, get good and angry.   —WILLIAM SAROYAN

✴

The proper function of man is to live, not to exist. I shall not waste my days in trying to prolong them. —JACK LONDON

✤

Once you accept your own death, all of a sudden you're free to live. You no longer care about your reputation. You no longer care except so far as your life can be used tactically —to promote a cause you believe in.
—SAUL ALINSKY

✤

Those who welcome death have only tried it from the ears up. —WILSON MIZNER

✤

Don't be afraid your life will end; be afraid it will never begin. —GRACE HANSEN

✤

Live, so you do not have to look back and say, "God, how I have wasted by life!"
—ELISABETH KÜBLER-ROSS

✤

The fear of death is more to be dreaded than death itself. —Publilius Syrus

The wise man looks at death with honesty, dignity and calm, recognizing that the tragedy it brings is inherent in the great gift of life.

—Corliss Lamont

It's not that I'm afraid to die. I just don't want to be there when it happens.

—Woody Allen

I am not going to fight against death but for life. —Norbert Segard

Time is lost when we have not lived a full life, time enriched by experience, creative endeavor, enjoyment, and suffering.

—Dietrich Bonhoeffer

Death is not the greatest loss in life. The greatest loss is what dies inside us while we live. —Norman Cousins

❧

What a wonderful life I've had. I only wish I'd realized it sooner. —Colette

❧

How old would you be if you didn't know how old you were? —Satchel Paige

❧

The bitterest tears shed over graves are for words left unsaid and deeds left undone. —Thomas Carlyle

❧

The measure of a man's life is the well spending of it, not the length. —Plutarch

❧

A long life lived is not good enough, but a good life lived is long enough. —Bernard Jensen

❧

As long as you're useful, you'll never be old.
—Leo F. Buscaglia

✶

You can't turn back the clock, but you can wind it up again. —Bonnie Prudden

✶

The secret of staying young is to live honestly, eat slowly, and lie about your age.
—Lucille Ball

✶

Don't let life discourage you; everyone who got where he is had to begin where he was.
—Richard Evans

✶

Don't fret over what you'd do with your time if you could live over again. . . . Get busy with what you have left. —Anonymous

✶

Not the power to remember, but the power to forget, is a necessary condition for our existence. —Sholem Asch

What lies behind us and what lies before us are tiny matters compared to what lies within us. —RALPH WALDO EMERSON

❧

Dost thou love life? Then do not squander time; for that's the stuff life is made of.
—BENJAMIN FRANKLIN

❧

May you live all the days of your life.
—JONATHAN SWIFT

❧

We must always change, renew, rejuvenate ourselves; otherwise we harden. —GOETHE

❧

Life is like a ten-speed bike. Most of us have gears we never use. —CHARLES M. SCHULTZ

❧

What I admire in Columbus is not his having discovered a world but having gone to search for it on the faith of an opinion.
—ANNE-ROBERT-JACQUES TURGOT

He who has a why to live can bear almost any how. —FRIEDRICH NIETZSCHE

❧

Life is not merely to be alive, but to be well. —MARTIAL

❧

Die, my dear doctor, is the last thing I shall do. —HENRY JOHN, LORD PALMERSTON

❧

If I'd known I was going to live so long, I'd have taken better care of myself.

—LEON ELDRED

❧

If one advances confidently in the direction of his dreams, and endeavors to live the life which he has imagined, he will meet with a success unexpected in common hours.

—HENRY DAVID THOREAU

❧

Where the road bends abruptly, take short steps. —ERNEST BRAMAB

✲

Where there is life there is hope. —CICERO

✲

This is our purpose: to make as meaningful as possible this life that has been bestowed upon us; to live in such a way that we may be proud of ourselves; to act in such a way that some part of us lives on. —OSWALD SPENGLER

✲

Life is not a trip itself. It's not a goal. It is a process. You get there step by step. And if every step is wondrous, and every step is magical, that's what life will be.

—LEO F. BUSCAGLIA

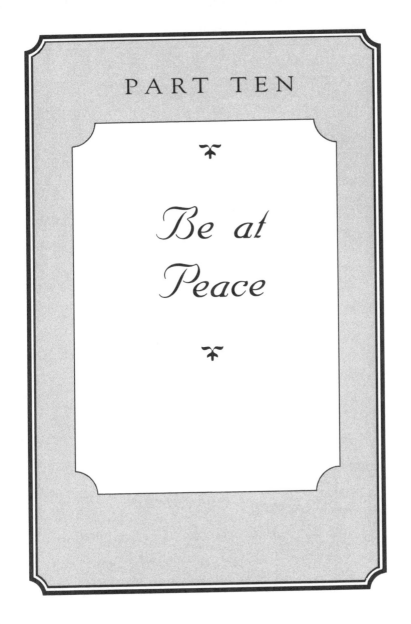

PART TEN

Be at

Peace

Take rest; a field that has rested gives a boun-
tiful crop.   —OVID

❋

To do nothing is sometimes a good remedy.
                              —HIPPOCRATES

❋

A quiet mind cureth all.   —ROBERT BURTON

❋

The thoughtful soul to solitude retires.
                              —OMAR KHAYYAM

❋

Pain is hard to bear. . . . But with patience,
day by day, even this shall pass away.
                              —THEODORE TILTON

❋

How poor are they who have not patience.
What wound did ever heal but by degrees?
                              —SHAKESPEARE

❋

For peace of mind, resign as general manager
of the universe.   —LARRY EISENBERG

Nothing can bring you peace but yourself.
                              —RALPH WALDO EMERSON

By a tranquil mind I mean nothing else than
a mind well ordered.   —MARCUS AURELIUS

I atrribute my long life to inward calm.
                              —CHINESE PROVERB

All human wisdom is summed up in two
words—wait and hope.
                              —ALEXANDRE DUMAS

Monotony is the law of nature. Look at the
monotonous manner in which the sun rises.
The monotony of necessary occupations is ex-
hilarating and life-giving.
                              —MAHATMA GANDHI

Healthful, soothing slumber that rests muscles, nerves, and brain is one of nature's greatest rejuvenators. —HARVEY DIAMOND

The best cure for insomnia is to get a lot of sleep. —W. C. FIELDS

My handicap is part of me because I have had to make peace with it. And in doing so, I've made peace with the less obvious handicaps of other people, like resentment, prejudice, hate. —GINGER HUTTON

Give yourself a few minutes every day to sit in quiet meditation. . . . Observe your breathing and allow the thoughts to pass gently through your mind. —LOUISE HAY

Rule number one is: "Don't sweat the small stuff." Rule number two is: "It's all small stuff." If you can't fight and you can't flee, flow. —ROBERT S. ELIOT

In the West, where the meditative tradition is not strong and people are not in the habit of stopping periodically to become quiet and reevaluate their lives, illness stops a person so he can step back and have an opportunity to take stock of what is important to him.

—MARTIN L. ROSSMAN

❧

Meditation is not a means to an end. It is both the means and the end.   —J. KRISHNAMURTI

❧

It is as important to relax our minds as it is to concentrate them.

—CHARLES B. NEWCOMB

❧

There is more to life than increasing its speed.

—MAHATMA GANDHI

❧

The trouble with the rat race is that even if you win, you're still a rat.   —LILY TOMLIN

❧

Humor, the ability to laugh at life, is right at the top, with love and communication, in the hierarchy of our needs. Humor has much to do with pain; it exaggerates the anxieties and absurdities we feel, so that we gain distance, and through laughter, relief.

—SARA DAVIDSON

❧

Laughter is a form of internal jogging. It moves your internal organs around. It enhances respiration. It is an igniter of great expectations.

—NORMAN COUSINS

❧

Laughter is a tranquilizer with no side effects.

—ARNOLD GLASOW

❧

He who laughs, lasts.

—MARY PETTIBONE POOLE

❧

Seriousness is a fatal disease.

—PAUL ZAMARIAN

❧

Just for today, I will have a program. I might not follow it exactly, but I will have it. I will save myself from two enemies—hurry and indecision.   —ALCOHOLICS ANONYMOUS

❦

STEPS TO RELIEVE STRESS

Talk it out. When something worries you, don't bottle it up. *Escape for a while.* When things go wrong, it helps to escape from the painful problem for a while. *Work off your anger.* Do something constructive with the pent-up energy. Pitch into some physical activity or work it out in tennis or a long walk. *Do something for others.* If you feel yourself worrying about yourself all the time, try doing something for somebody else. *Take one thing at a time.* Take a few of the most urgent tasks and pitch into them, one at a time, setting aside all the rest for the time being. *Shun the "superman" urge.* No one can be perfect in everything.

—NATIONAL MENTAL HEALTH ASSOCIATION

❦

It is a happy talent to know how to play.
                    —RALPH WALDO EMERSON

By working faithfully eight hours a day you may eventually get to be boss and work twelve hours a day. —ROBERT FROST

☥

Sitting quietly by oneself and being aware of all that's taking place in the mind and body can lead to rejuvenation. —STAN LIPKEN

☥

In those few moments [of meditation] when the mind becomes calm, we experience a peacefulness, a contentment that is the inner self, the part of our consciousness that is not conditioned by past experience.

—JOAN BORYSENKO

☥

Healing perspective: My dad believed in meditation. . . . He used to tell me, "Sit down and shut up." —BILL DANA

☥

It is certain that the personality without conflict is immune from illness.

—EDWARD BACH

If we can only set aside a short time every day, quite alone and in as quiet a place as possible, free from interruption, and merely sit or lie quietly, either keeping the mind blank or calmly thinking of one's walk in life, it will be found after a time that we get great help at such moments and, as it were, flashes of knowledge and guidance are given to us. We find the questions of the difficult problems of life are unmistakably answered, and we become able to choose with confidence the right course. —EDWARD BACH

It is universally admitted that there is a natural healing power resident in the body. . . . Many people have learned to relax and keep quiet like the animals, giving nature a free opportunity to heal their maladies.

—HORATIO W. DRESSER

Simplify, simplify.

—HENRY DAVID THOREAU

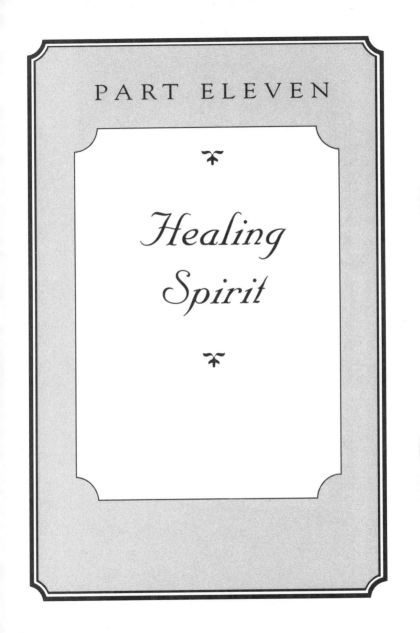

PART ELEVEN

Healing
Spirit

The Serenity Prayer
God grant me the serenity to accept
the things I cannot change,
courage to change the things I can,
and the wisdom to know the
difference.   —Reinhold Niebuhr

꙳

I would rather walk with God in the dark than
go alone in the light.
—Mary Gardiner Brainard

꙳

Never think that God's delays are God's denials. Hold on; hold fast; hold out. Patience is
genius.   —Comte de Buffon

꙳

In my soul I know that God knows me and
loves me, and loves me even though he knows
me. My heart has every reason to smile.
—Greg Anderson

꙳

Of course God will forgive me; that's his
business.   —Lorenz Oken

Love is very patient and kind, never jealous or envious, never boastful or proud, never haughty or selfish or rude. Love does not demand its own way. It is not irritable or touchy. It does not hold grudges and will hardly even notice when others do it wrong. It is never glad about injustice, but rejoices whenever truth wins out. There are three things that remain—faith, hope, and love—and the greatest of these is love.　　—SAINT PAUL

❋

Afflictions are but the shadow of God's wings.
　　　　　　　　　—GEORGE MACDONALD

❋

Let us not be justices of the peace but angels of peace.　　—SAINTE THÉRÈSE DE LISIEUX

❋

Let your light so shine before men that they may see your good works and glorify your father which is in heaven.

—SAINT MATTHEW

❋

God is with us in the darkness as surely as he is with us in the light.   —*Our Daily Bread*

❧

Lord, make me an instrument of your peace. Where there is hatred, let me sow love; where there is injury, pardon; where there is doubt, faith; where there is despair, hope; where there is darkness, light; and where there is sadness, joy.   —SAINT FRANCIS OF ASSISI

❧

More things are wrought by prayer than this world dreams of.

—ALFRED, LORD TENNYSON

❧

The light of God surrounds me;
The love of God enfolds me;
The power of God protects me;
The presence of God watches over me.
Wherever I am, God is.

—JAMES DILLET FREEMAN

❧

The earnest prayer of a righteous man has great power and wonderful results.

—Saint James

❋

The value of persistent prayer is not that he will hear us, but that we will finally hear him.

—William McGill

❋

He who abandons himself to God will never be abandoned by God.   —*Our Daily Bread*

❋

Walk with God and you'll always reach your destination.   —Anonymous

❋

We cannot go where God is not, and where God is, all is well.   —Anonymous

❋

Yea, though I walk through the valley of the shadow of death, I will fear no evil: for thou art with me; thy rod and thy staff they comfort me.   —*Psalm 23*

May I seek to live this day
    quietly, serenely
leaning on your mighty strength
    trustfully, restfully
meeting others in the path
    peacefully, joyously
waiting for your will's unfolding
    patiently, obediently
facing what tomorrow brings
    confidently, courageously.
        —ANONYMOUS

❧

Faith is a living and unshakeable confidence,
a belief in the grace of God.
        —MARTIN LUTHER

❧

Love God and trust your feelings. Be loyal to
them. Don't betray them.
        —ROBERT POLLACK

❧

God is love, but get it in writing.
        —GYPSY ROSE LEE

❧

Our spiritual lives are strengthened as we find that precious balance between expectant trust in our higher power and responsible reliance on ourselves. —SEFRA PITZELE

Never give up. This may be your moment for a miracle. —GREG ANDERSON

True miracles are created by men where they use the courage and intelligence that God gave them. —JEAN ANNILK

Call on God but row away from the rocks. —INDIAN PROVERB

If you will only help yourself, God will help you. —MATHURIN RÉGNIER

Whatever your job, it is important if it is what God wants you to do. —HENRY JACOBSEN

God's love does not exempt us from trials but sees us through them.   —*Our Daily Bread*

❉

Faith is not shelter against difficulties but belief in the face of all contradictions.

—PAUL TOURNIER

❉

Healing seldom appears from heaven. It comes in a kit. Assembly is required.

—ANONYMOUS

❉

Slow me down, Lord. . . . Teach me the art of taking minute vacations.   —ORIN CRANE

❉

I treated him, God cured him.

—AMBROISE PAR

❉

It is for us to make the effort. The result is always in God's hands.

—MAHATMA GANDHI

❉

What we are is God's gift to us. What we become is our gift to God. —Louis Nizer

❧

The real purpose of attaining better physical health and longer life is not just the enjoyment of a pain- and disease-free existence, but a higher divine purpose for which life was given to us. —Paavo O. Airola

❧

Whatever things are true, whatever things are noble, whatever things are just, whatever things are pure, whatever things are lovely, whatever things are of good report, if there is any virtue and if there is anything praiseworthy—meditate on these things.

—Saint Paul

❧

I've heard He works with broken people. I am sick, hurting, broken. I am waiting and willing now. —Flora E. Meredith

❧

Fear imprisons, faith liberates;
Fear paralyzes, faith empowers;
Fear disheartens, faith encourages;
Fear sickens, faith heals;
Fear makes useless, faith makes
    serviceable.
       —HARRY EMERSON FOSDICK

Feed your faith and your doubts will starve to
death.   —*Sparks From the Anvil*

O my soul, don't be discouraged. Don't be upset. Expect God to act.   —*Psalms*

When you have nothing left but God, you become aware that God is enough.
              —*Guideposts*

Walk softly.
Speak tenderly.
Pray fervently.
  —ANONYMOUS

Prayer is not asking. It is a longing of the soul.
—MAHATMA GANDHI

Faith has a powerful effect in helping people recover a sense of balance, tranquility, and hope.
—ROBERT VENINGA

Joy is the echo of God's life within us.
—JOSEPH MARION

Our goal is peace—
with self,
with others,
with God.
—GREG ANDERSON